Overview

Topic:

The Ultimate Guide on Becoming Your Best Version by Living a Life of Wellness

Introduction

- Why we are talking about becoming your best version and Wellness
- Who this post is for
- Why is wellness important
- What is Wellness
- Behaviors that promote wellness (how to live a life of wellness)

- What is Wellness (and Why Does it Matter)

The Benefits of Wellness

- *All the great things about Wellness*

Behaviors that promote wellness

- The way that you behave when you are on a path of wellness

Closing

Call-to-Action

The Ultimate Guide on Becoming Your Best Version by Living a Life of Wellness

Do you want to achieve more in your life? Are you thinking about how to make more money, sleep better, maintain relationships, and be happier? Everyone wants to be a high achiever and you can become your best version in a matter of time by living a life of wellness. If your answer to the previous questions were yes, this post is for you. According to Total Access Medical "Wellness is a conscious, self-directed and evolving process of achieving full potential."

I believe that you can start improving your life today by changing what you eat. We are what we eat and I have seen myself have more energy and vigor when I consume a clean and delicious meal. Man, I'm telling you! Great food topped off with exercise, opens up the doors to living a life where I am in control. I'm not perfect, this is why I do my best when I am attempting anything in life.

I make a conscious effort to love myself and others, I always encourage my friends and family to eat right, exercise, take time for themselves, and challenge themselves, etc. I just want what's best for the people around me so we can all live well and this is why I am sharing this guide with you.

In this guide you will understand:

- What is wellness and why it matters?
- Behaviors that promote wellness.
- The benefits of wellness.
- Components of Wellness.

1. WHAT IS WELLNESS AND WHY IT MATTERS?

Wellness is to consistently make the most of each moment and consciously chose to live a better life each day. Brheadstart.org states that "It is important for everyone to achieve optimal wellness in order to subdue stress, reduce the risk of illness and ensure positive interactions." We can save ourselves a lot of trouble by putting our priorities first.

Let's talk about the dimensions of wellness, I've heard that there are 9, 8, 7 and sometimes 12 dimensions of wealth. Today we will stick to 5. According to Roger Williams University, there are 5 dimensions of wealth which are:

- Physical:

This includes the overall physical state of the body, inside and out. This is a mixture of good eating habits, regular exercise, sleeping enough, having balance in terms of what the body consumes and does physically. In order to maintain good physical health it is necessary to get 6-8 hours of sleep each night, eat meals on time, avoid overeating. It is also important to have respect for your surroundings and yourself, maintain a clean body and environment. The connection between health, emotional balance and physical well-being, however, has so far been undisputed. But what exactly is it now? Like health, well-being is a state of mind and body. If nothing is missing in the body and the psyche, then we are healthy, and our well-being is unaffected. This is the optimal state that we humans perceive as positive and pleasant psychologically, which we - often only unconsciously - want to maintain or just want to bring about again.

Pain, illness and other health and physical restrictions can affect our well-being. However, the good news is that we significantly influence our general well-being through our diet and lifestyle. More and more people want to be active not only for a slim appearance or their health but also for physical well-being in general. With exercise such as walking, walking the dog or endurance sports such as swimming or cycling, we enjoy ourselves all around.

Sleep provides relaxation and even slows down aging processes. The brain and body work at full speed at night: A high concentration of growth hormones ensures that stored metabolic products are broken down, and injuries in the body tissue are healed. To maintain and strengthen general physical well-being, more and more people are becoming active themselves. Conventional medicine is no longer the only factor when it comes to our well-being! A balanced diet makes a significant contribution to a healthy lifestyle and forms the basis of your well-being. The food should provide your body with all the vital substances it needs for a strong nervous and immune system. The essential factors of a healthy lifestyle show that a holistic definition of health must include both the body and the psyche.

- Emotional:

This includes maintaining control over emotions, taking time to respond to situations maturely. Taking time for yourself and to know who you truly are. It is difficult to achieve self-actualization if you don't know who you truly are. Having a positive outlook on life and choosing to be happy contributes greatly to your health. It is essential to work on our emotional health in order to decrease stress levels. Emotional and physical health is two sides of the same coin, and maintaining our emotional well-being is critical to leading healthy and fulfilling lives.
Current research has been taken on emotional well-being. This defines well-being in terms of happiness, positive affect, low negative affect, and life satisfaction, while the eudemonic perspective emphasizes positive psychological functioning, optimal

experience, and development. As a rule, it is assumed that emotional well-being is multidimensional and not equated with happiness or the absence of suffering and disturbances. Emotional Well-being can be divided into subjective, psychological and social well-being and described using various elements.

Emotional well-being focuses on personal growth and self-realization. It is defined as the extent to which a person is fully functional. It includes, among other things, the exhaustion of your potential and the fulfilment of your own "true nature". When you can act independently in your life, master environmental demands, experience personal development, sustain healthy relationships with others, understand the meaning in life, and embrace yourself; you have a high degree of emotional well-being.

Social togetherness and relationships are essential aspects of life, and people actively seek emotional and physical interactions with other people. Healthy relationships can hold up and be a source of joy in difficult times. Success, performance and competence are sought for their own sake and also contribute to emotional well-being.

- Social:

Interact with others, form bonds and different types of relationships. Bring value to the people around you, stay active in your community and play your part in improving whatever you can with your skills. Work on improving your communication skills, limit time with negative or toxic people. Be honest, love yourself and set a good example. Practice good qualities in private so that you behave well in public. Be a blessing to the world and not a nuisance. People do a lot for their health: ideally, they reduce their tobacco consumption, drink less alcohol, eat a balanced diet and do more sport. But what also plays a unique role for the human psyche is often neglected: mental health. From a social perspective, the topic is now being taken up and interpreted in different ways. For example, the range of social media channels is only an indication of the human need to network and communicate. Of course, personal contacts and friendships come first and satisfy the basic need from birth: to feel that we belong.

Many times, social interactions have been clinically shown to have a huge effect on our emotional well-being. Loneliness and the lack of social ties can even make you sick in the long run. It has been proven that this isolation is comparable to the physical damage that occurs when smoking 15 cigarettes a day, for example. In addition, recent researches show that a lack of social connection is twice as alarming as obesity.

The influence of social contacts has a significant effect on your well-being - if it is the right contacts for you. They strengthen your immune system and protect against depression or other mental illnesses. They also improve the way you deal with stress and thereby improve your heart and circulation at the same time.

It may not be accessible in the hustle and bustle of everyday working life - but time for your family and friends is good and valuable time invested. You will notice: Not only you but also your (real) joys will be better in the long term.

- Spiritual:

Make time to reflect on your life, think about all the great things and people you have attracted in your life, visualize and believe in your aspirations. Forgive the people that did you wrong in the past and forgive yourself for the mistakes you have made. Take time to be aware of your daily actions, live in the present moment and ask for guidance. A spiritual journey encourages self assessment and appreciation for your life. It all comes down to balancing body, mind, feelings, and spirit and encouraging health well-being when it comes to enjoying everyday life. By making small and continuous efforts every day, everyone can live a happier life.

Here are five simple spiritual wellness tips that will transform your life and encourage you to live completely every day.

Meditate
Although we cannot see or feel stress, it has a profound effect on
many people. Tension raises blood pressure and accelerates the heart
rate for a short period of time. Stress has a long-term detrimental
effect on the immune system, brain activity, and other vital organs.

One of the ideal ways to deal with stress is to meditate for 20 to 30
minutes a day. Meditation relaxes spiritual well-being. Meditation
regularly can also help keep chronic stress away. Meditation, in
numerous ways, may help to calm the mind, body, and spirit.
Meditation increases insight, imagination, and relation to the inner
self by influencing the sympathetic nervous system.

Spend time outdoors
So many people spend their working days cooped up indoors, with
no time to enjoy the outdoors. In the long term, this can have a lot of
adverse effects. A deficit of sunlight and fresh air can affect the
immune system, leading to chronic illness. Go for a walk at least 30
minutes a day to relax your mind and soul. It's good to give a break
to your routine and go on a trip to relax and enjoy.

Listen to good music.
When it comes to emotional well-being, music has always been an
enjoyable therapy.
Although music's effects are still not adequately understood,
research has found that music positively impacts one's spiritual well-
being.

Dopamine (it is a type of neurotransmitter) is emitted when you
listen to music. This is a chemical that elevates one's mood while
lowering anxiety and stress. Additionally, music can assist in
enhancing cognition and memory, helping you to exercise more
effectively.

Break your routine
While maintaining a routine and sticking to schedules is suitable for
your health. Breaking routines is a welcome change for the mind and
body. Of course, not everyone can break their routines at will. Don't

waste time; if you break your routine, you will like it. This will revive and keep you in a better mood.

Make love
Last but not least, loving your life partner can also benefit your health and well-being. It is a proven fact that the health benefits of lovemaking extend beyond the walls of the bedroom. Love boosts the immune system, lowers blood pressure, reduces acne, promotes better sleep, relieves stress and anxiety, and reduces heart disease risk.

- Intellectual:

  In order to become your best self it is important to keep learning. Ask questions, do research, read and exercise your brain. The more you use your brain, the easier it will be to use it. If there is something your good at, grow your knowledge in the field and become an expert. Make use of media and analyze trends. There is always something to learn. "Knowledge has a beginning but no end" – Gaeta Lyengar

2. BEHAVIOURS THAT PROMOTE WELLNESS (HOW TO LIVE A LIFE OF WELLNESS?)

What we do in each day determines the life we live as time goes by. By living a life of wellness, you have to live well even when no one is looking. It's in the way you carry yourself, how you spend your days, how you treat yourself, how you treat problems in life.

Be a healthy eater and exercise

A great life starts first thing each morning with what you eat and what you do with your body. What you eat determines your progress throughout the day, how you solve problems and how you think. If you start your day eating unhealthy food it's highly likely that you would want to continue on that path. Eating junk can slow down your pace in terms of thinking and physical movement.

Be a heathy eater and maintain a clean diet with regular exercise or else you will find yourself lacking on the energy you need to make the right decisions and put your priorities first. Let me give you an example; here is Joe, a supervisor and father of 2 newborn babies. Joe does his best to wake up early in the morning for work to exercise. All of his meals for the week were already packed in the fridge from over the weekend, all of his outfits for the week were pressed and ready to wear.

He eats a balanced diet everyday with no greasy food and his only source of sweets are usually from fruits or sweet potatoes, this is a fine example of someone that maintains a good diet and is full of energy. Joe is always on time for work, helps his team successfully meet deadlines, exceed expectations and Joe is always home early to help his wife take care of the children 50% of the time.

Manage yourself well

Living a life of wellness includes managing your time well so that you have enough time to sleep, getting enough sleep gives your body enough time to recover from vigorous exercises, and you have a stronger immune system when you get enough sleep. It is easier to speak with the people around you, be loving and empathetic when you get enough rest.

A true wellness journey never involves rushing to get things done therefore when you manage your time well, you can work comfortably and think clearly. You procrastinate less and understand how to ignore distractions.

Great management skills helps us not to overindulge on activities such as drinking, spending money, sleeping too long, eating too much and so on. You tend to know your limits and no when to stop. This is essential for having success in life.

Be Positive

Make an effort to be positive about your life. Always remember to be grateful and make the most out of what you have. A life of wellness helps you to attract more when you are positive. Positivity leads to an open mind. Be open to growth, try new things. If you never try, you will never know if something is for you, the possibilities are endless when you try new things.

Be Determined

Always push yourself and be willing to go the extra mile to do what many think is unbelievable. Believe in yourself and motivate yourself to achieve your goals in life. True wellness comes with great determination and a need to do the things you said you would. Success begins with wellness, as a matter of fact, wellness is success itself. When you embark on a journey of wellness you discover a perspective on life that allows you to see what it is that you need to do in order to achieve your goals. Never give up and press on with any challenge you face, you come out stronger and place yourself in a better position to do better the next time you end up in a tough situation.

3. THE BENEFITS OF WELLNESS

The benefits are endless when you begin your wellness journey, You can expect physical, emotional, social, spiritual and intellectual benefits.

The physical benefits include a higher life expectancy, improvement in physical appearance due to good nutrition and exercise. The process of aging is also decreased therefore you will have less wrinkles, plump skin, toned muscles and an overall more attractive demeanor. Be sure to expect an increase in energy and stamina as well

As for the emotional benefits of a wellness lifestyle, you will find that you have more control over the situations you face in life. You will feel an enhanced level of confidence and work well under pressure.

The social benefits of a wellness lifestyle improves how well you associate and communicate with others. This has major benefits in your career life and how you make deals. Great social skills propel high achievers to promotions at work. Long lasting relationships is a must and you will be seen as a trust worthy person that others can count on.

Some spiritual benefits include the ability to trust your intuition and manifest your vision for life. It is easier to accept yourself and to be honest with yourself when you maintain a wellness lifestyle. People with a clean heart usually attract good spirited people around them and have less stress in their lives. You can easily make yourself happy, control your anger and live a life of peace even when you face obstacles in your life.

Faster thinking, ability to solve problems accurately and rapidly, highly informed and have the ability to teach others very well; these are some of the benefits of being intellectual. You would have the ability to take on large amount of tasks and find a smart way to complete them. People living on the intellectual side of life have a higher chance to make more money in a shorter period of time because of how educated they are.

If you are intellectual, people usually look up to you and are quickly willing to offer you help when you're in need. This wellness trait also comes with the ability to organize well whether it be your physical space or your mind. Living a life of wellness can improve memory and help you to avoid terrible diseases or illnesses. An intellectual mind knows how to quickly overcome problems when they find themselves in a bad position.

In Conclusion, when you make up your mind to work every day towards your overall success in life you achieve more. We must do our best to maintain good wellness habits in order to increase our ability to successfully take on challenges and win. We need to make the most of each moment in our lives.

Leave us a comment and share with us how you live a life of wellness.

References:

William Kirkpatrick., What is Wellness & Why Is It Important? - Total Access Medical 2021; Available from: http://wellness.totalaccessmedical.com/blog/what-is-wellness#:~:text=Wellness%20matters%20because%20everything%20we,affects%20our%20actions%20and%20emotions.&text=Therefore%2C%20it%20is%20important%20for,illness%20and%20ensure%20positive%20interactions.

N.A., Mental Health and Wellness.docx- Brheadstart n.d; Available from: http://www.brheadstart.org/wp-content/uploads/2013/10/Mental-Health-and-Wellness.pdf

N.A., Roger Williams University 2021; Available from: https://www.rwu.edu/undergraduate/student-life/health-and-counseling/health-education-program/dimensions-wellness

Geeta Lyengar., Johann Goethe's 'Knowledge Has A Beginning But No End' – IPL 2021; Available from:

60 Recipes For a Healthier Living

Vegan

1. **Avocado and smoked tofu toast**: Ingredients: 0.5 zucchini, 1 tofu, 1/4 cup soy sauce, 2 ounces garlic powder, 2 ounces smoked paprika powder, 1 avocado, 3,8 ounces sliced almonds   Marinade tofu and zucchini slices in soy sauce, garlic powder, and smoked paprika powder, then heat in a fry pan with some oil. Place avocado, tofu and zucchini, and sliced almonds on a piece of toast and enjoy! (1 portion) (15min)

2. **Tofu-fruit smoothie**: Ingredients:0,8 cups frozen blueberries, 0,5 cup unsweetened almond milk, walnuts, 0,5 avocado, 1/4 cup frozen strawberries, 0.5 frozen banana Put the ingredients into the blender and blend until smooth and creamy!

3. **Scrambled tofu:** Ingredients: 1 tablespoon olive oil, bunch of green onions, chopped, couple of cherry tomatoes, 1 package firm silken tofu, drained and mashed, ground turmeric to taste, salt and pepper to taste Heat olive oil in a medium skillet over medium heat, and sauté green onions until tender. Cut tomatoes in half. Stir in tomatoes and mashed tofu. Season with salt, pepper, and turmeric. Reduce heat, and simmer until heated through. (1 portion) (15min)

4. **Baked tofu with broccoli:** Ingredients: 1 package extra firm tofu, 1 large broccoli, cut up, 2 tablespoon olive oil, 2 ounces garlic powder, 1 tablespoon cornstarch or arrowroot powder, 1 cup freshly squeezed orange juice (or grapefruit),

0,5 cup sliced green onion, bunch of fresh cilantro
Preheat oven to 392 degrees. Drain the tofu cut it into 1-2
inch cubes. In a large mixing bowl whisk together 15ml
olive oil, garlic powder. Marinate the tofu in the mixture
until all of the liquid is almost all absorbed, this should
take just a few minutes. Sprinkle with cornstarch and toss
lightly. Line two baking sheets with parchment paper and
spray them lightly with the olive oil spray. Distribute the
tofu on one and the broccoli on the other. Sprinkle the
broccoli with sea salt and a touch more olive oil. Pop them
both in the oven, the tofu on the rack nearest the bottom
and the broccoli on the top. Roast for 20 - 25 minutes, and
flipping the tofu and broccoli halfway through. The tofu
should be golden brown and crispy on both sides and the
broccoli should be bright green and just starting to brown.
Drizzle the orange juice onto the tofu. (1-2 portion)
(40min)

5. **Spicy tempeh:** Ingredients: 1 package tempeh, chopped
   into 2.5cm cubes, 1 yellow onion, 2 chopped kales, 1
   avocado, 2 tablespoon olive oil, 0, 5 cup freshly squeezed
   lime juice, 4 cloves garlic, minced, 1 tbsp. minced ginger, 1
   tablespoon honey, 2 ounces nutmeg, 2 ounces cumin, 2
   ounces cinnamon, 1 ounce cayenne pepper, salt to taste, 2
   cups rice/quinoa/lentils etc. Mix together the ingredients in
   a medium bowl. In a second large bowl, add the tempeh and
   onion and pour the marinade over -making sure to cover all
   the pieces. Cover and refrigerate overnight or at least 3
   hours. Cook grain according to package directions and have
   warmed when ready to serve. When ready to cook, heat a
   tablespoon of olive in a large skillet over medium high heat
   and then add the marinated tempeh and all additional

liquid. Cook for at least 5 minutes or until the majority of the liquid has cooked off. Add kale and cook for 5 additional minutes -making sure to stir the dish. When ready to serve, serve the tempeh over the grain and add avocado to garnish and enjoy! (1-2 portion) (30min)

6. **Lemon- garlic tempeh:** Ingredients: 1 package of tempeh, sliced into strips, 4 cloves of garlic, minced, 1 tablespoon olive oil, 0,5 ounces freshly minced ginger, 0,5 ounces cumin, 1 cup of kale, 1 lemons' juice
Place chopped kale in boiling water for 3 minutes. Remove with a slotted spoon and place the kale in a bowl of ice water. Drain well. You may have to actually squeeze the kale to wring out all the extra liquid. Heat olive oil in a large skillet over medium heat. Add tempeh strips and cook for 2-3 minutes, flip and cook for another 2 minutes or until both sides of the tempeh slices are brown. Meanwhile tempeh is browning, whisk together the lemon juice, garlic, ginger and cumin in a small bowl. Once tempeh has browned, add kale and the lemony garlic mixture. Stir to coat. Cook for 2-3 minutes. Remove the heat, add salt and ground pepper to taste and serve. (1 portion) (20min)

7. **Tempeh with vegetables and quinoa:** Ingredients: 1 package tempeh, 1 tablespoon olive oil, bunch of fresh coriander, couple of stems of asparagus, 0,5 cup cooked black beans, 0,5 cup cooked quinoa, 5 cherry tomatoes, 3 ounces curry powder, 4 ounces of salsa   Heat olive oil in a medium skillet over medium heat. Add the tempeh, stir fry until golden brown and add your vegetables, spices and salsa until cooked and browned. Sprinkle with coriander or with other fresh herbs and serve. (1 portion) (30min)

Fish

(Fish is easier to digest than chicken and beef and it has lots of protein value)

8. **garlic salmon:** Ingredients: 1 1/2 pounds salmon fillet, salt and pepper to taste, 3 cloves garlic, minced, 1 sprig fresh dill, chopped, 5 slices lemon, 5 sprigs fresh dill weed, 2 green onions, chopped   Preheat oven to 450 degrees F. Spray two large pieces of aluminum foil with cooking spray. Place salmon fillet on top of one piece of foil. Sprinkle salmon with salt, pepper, garlic and chopped dill. Arrange lemon slices on top of fillet and place a sprig of dill on top of each lemon slice. Sprinkle fillet with chopped scallions. Cover salmon with second piece of foil and pinch together foil to tightly seal. Place on a baking sheet or in a large baking dish. Bake in preheated oven for 20-25 minutes, until salmon flakes easily. (fish)

9. **Tuna steak with baked sweet potatoes:** Ingredients: 3 medium sized sweet potatoes, salt, pepper, teaspoon of olive oil, tuna fillet   Skin and cut the sweet potatoes, salt them and bake them in the oven on 180 Celsius until they are soft. Heat up a grilling pan, add a drop of olive oil and place in the tuna which you can season optionally but I recommend simply salt and pepper. Grill it till the outside becomes light pink and a bit burned, than take it out. (fish)

10. **Canned tuna with avocado and steamed broccoli (tuna salad):** Ingredients: 1 broccoli, 1 can of tuna, 1 avocado Boil water than add sea salt and cut broccoli. Boil the broccoli till

it becomes soft but do not overcook! Open a can of tuna, take the fish out, take off the skin and cut an avocado. Mix the ingredients and tuna salad is done. (fish)

11. **garlic-lemon tilapia :** Ingredients: 4 tilapia fillets, 3 tablespoons fresh lemon juice, 1 tablespoon butter, melted, 1 clove garlic, finely chopped, 1 teaspoon dried parsley flakes, pepper to taste   Preheat oven to 380 degrees F . Spray a baking dish with non-stick cooking spray. Place fillets in the baking dish. Pour lemon juice over fillets, and then drizzle butter on top. Sprinkle with garlic, parsley, and pepper. Bake in preheated oven until the fish is white and flakes when pulled apart with a fork, about 30-35 minutes. (fish)

12. **salmon steak with couscous:** Ingredients: 1 salmon fillet, salt, 2 cups of water, 2 cups of couscous, ground black pepper, slices of lemon   Sprinkle the salmon fillets with a little salt. Place salmon fillets, skin-side down on the pan. Cover. Cook 5 to 10 minutes, depending on the thickness of the fillet. Do not overcook. Bring 2 cups water to boil in a pot. Remove from heat, and mix in couscous. Cover, and let sit 5 minutes. Serve the cooked salmon over couscous, and drizzle with sauce from skillet. Serve the dish sprinkled with freshly ground black pepper and a slice or two of lemon. (fish)

13. **Salmon steak with steamed asparagus:** Ingredients: 1tbsp olive oil, 3 cloves garlic, ¼ cup water, 1 tbsp. lemon juice, salt and pepper, bunch of cherry tomatoes, cilantro, 1 salmon fillet   Heat the olive oil in a large skillet over medium heat. Place salmon in the skillet, and season with garlic, lemon pepper and salt. Pour water around salmon. Place tomatoes and cilantro in the skillet. Cover, and cook 15 minutes, or until fish is easily flaked with a fork. Heat a

pan on medium heat; add garlic, olive oil and asparagus. Cook it till it gets soft and enjoy the meal! (fish)

14. **Broiled tilapia:** Ingredients: 1/2 cup Parmesan cheese, 1/4 cup butter, softened, 2 tablespoons mayonnaise, 2 tablespoons fresh lemon juice, 1/4 teaspoon dried basil, 1/4 teaspoon ground black pepper, 1/8 teaspoon onion powder, salt, 2 pounds tilapia fillets   Preheat your oven's broiler. Grease a broiling pan or line pan with aluminum foil. In a small bowl, mix together the Parmesan cheese, butter, mayonnaise and lemon juice. Season with dried basil, pepper, onion powder and salt. Mix and set aside. Arrange fillets in a single layer on the prepared pan. Broil a few inches from the heat for 2 to 3 minutes. Flip the fillets over and broil for a couple more minutes. Remove the fillets from the oven and cover them with the Parmesan cheese mixture on the top side. Broil for 2 more minutes or until the topping is browned and fish flakes easily with a fork. Be careful not to overcook the fish. (fish, milk)

15. **Sesame seared tuna:** Ingredients: 1/4 cup soy sauce, 1 tablespoon mirin (Japanese sweet wine), 1 tablespoon honey, 2 tablespoons sesame oil, 1 tablespoon rice wine vinegar, 4 (6 ounce) tuna steaks, 1/2 cup sesame seeds, wasabi paste, 1 tablespoon olive oil,   In a small bowl, stir together the soy sauce, mirin, honey and sesame oil. Divide into two equal parts. Stir the rice vinegar into one part and set aside as a dipping sauce. Coat the tuna steaks with the remaining soy sauce mixture, then press into the sesame seeds to coat. Heat olive oil in a cast iron skillet over high heat until very hot. Place steaks in the pan, and sear for about 30 seconds on each side. Serve with the dipping sauce and wasabi paste if desired. (fish, soy)

16. **Pan seared tilapia:** Ingredients: 4 fillets tilapia, salt and pepper to taste, 1/2 cup all-purpose flour, 1 tablespoon olive oil, 2 tablespoons unsalted butter, melted

    Rinse tilapia fillets in cold water and pat dry with paper towels. Season both sides of each fillet with salt and pepper. Gently press each fillet into flour to coat and shake off the excess flour. Heat the olive oil in a skillet over medium-high heat; cook the tilapia in the hot oil until the fish flakes easily with a fork, about 4 minutes per side. Brush the melted butter onto the tilapia in the last minute before removing from the skillet. Serve immediately. (fish, wheat, milk)

17. **almond-tilapia:** Ingredients: 2 eggs, 1 teaspoon lemon pepper, 1 teaspoon garlic pepper, 1 cup ground almonds, 1 cup freshly grated Parmesan cheese, 8 (6 ounce) tilapia fillets, 1/4 cup all-purpose flour for dusting, 6 tablespoons butter, salt to taste, 1 cup freshly grated Parmesan cheese, 8 sprigs parsley, 8 lemon wedges   Beat the eggs with the lemon pepper and garlic pepper until blended; set aside. Stir together ground almonds with 1 cup of Parmesan cheese in a shallow dish until combined; set aside. Dust the tilapia fillets with flour, and shake off excess. Dip the tilapia in egg, then press into the almond mixture. Melt butter in a large skillet over medium-high heat. Cook tilapia in melted butter until golden brown on both sides, 2.5-3 minutes per side. Reduce heat to medium, and season fillets with salt if desired. Sprinkle the tilapia with the remaining Parmesan cheese, cover, and continue cooking until the Parmesan cheese has melted, about 5 minutes. Transfer the tilapia to a serving dish, and garnish with parsley springs to serve. (fish, tree nut, milk, wheat)

18. **Baked tilapia:** Ingredients: 2tbsp butter, 1 tbsp. lemon juice, 1 clove of garlic tilapia fillet, fresh parsley

Preheat an oven to 380 degrees F; prepare a baking dish with cooking spray. Combine the butter, lemon juice, and garlic in a bowl; heat in microwave in 10-second increments until the butter is completely melted and the garlic has softened, stirring between each session, about 1 minute total. Arrange the tilapia in the bottom of the prepared baking dish; pour the butter mixture over the fillets assuring they are all evenly covered. Sprinkle the parsley over the tilapia. Bake in the preheated oven, turning the fillets every 10 minutes, until the fish flakes easily with a fork, about 40 minutes total. (fish, milk)

19. **Sesame tilapia:** Ingredients: 2 (4 ounce) fillets tilapia, 1/4 cup sesame oil, 1 clove garlic, minced, salt to taste, fresh ground black pepper to taste
Place the tilapia in a bowl, and drizzle with the sesame oil. Season with the garlic, kosher salt, and pepper. Cover, and marinate at least 30 minutes in the refrigerator. Preheat oven to 355 degrees F. Transfer the tilapia and marinade to a baking dish, and bake 30-35 minutes in the preheated oven, until fish is easily flaked with a fork. (Fish)

20. **Ginger salmon:** Ingredients: 2 teaspoons olive oil, 1 tablespoon honey, 1 tablespoon Dijon mustard, 2 teaspoons grated fresh ginger, 1 pound salmon fillets   Preheat oven to 350 degrees F (175 degrees C). In a small bowl, blend olive oil, honey, Dijon mustard and ginger. Brush salmon fillets evenly with the olive oil mixture. Place in a medium baking dish. Bake 15 - 20 minutes in the preheated oven, until the fish flakes easily with a fork. (fish)

Egg

(Egg white contains the most protein compared to its size among all protein sources. Egg yolks contain a lot of good and healthy fats which is recommended to be consumed at the first meal of the day)

21. **Slice of whole-grain bread with avocado on it and poached egg on top:** Ingredients: a slice of whole grain bread, 1 avocado, vinegar, salt, 1 egg   Toast a slice of whole-grain bread than spread an avocado on it. Fill a saucepan with cold water and place over medium heat; stir in vinegar and salt. Bring to a gentle, slow simmer and reduce heat to low. Break each egg into a separate small ramekin; place a ramekin close to the surface of the water and gently pour egg into the simmering water. Let egg white set for a minute or two and use a silicone spatula to gently lift egg from the bottom of the pan to prevent sticking. Cook until white is firm and yolk is runny, about 6 minutes. Lift poached egg from water using a spoon and transfer gently to bowl of ice water to stop the cooking process. Reheat eggs for 0.5- 1.5 minutes in very gently simmering water and remove with a slotted spoon. Tap bottom of slotted spoon containing egg on a dry paper towel to remove the excess water before serving. Place the egg on top of your toast and enjoy! (egg, wheat)

22. **poached egg with asparagus:** Ingredients: 4 eggs, 1 pound fresh asparagus, trimmed, 4 slices whole wheat bread, 4 slices Cheddar cheese, 1 tablespoon butter, salt and pepper to taste   Fill a saucepan half way full of water and bring it to a boil .Crack one egg into a measuring cup or large spoon and gently slip it into the boiling water. Repeat with remaining eggs. Simmer for about 5 minutes over medium heat. Remove with a slotted spoon and keep warm.

Meanwhile, Place the asparagus into a saucepan and fill with enough water to cover. Bring to a boil, and cook until asparagus is tender, about 4 minutes then drain. Roast the bread to your desired darkness. Spread butter onto each piece of toast. Top with a slice of cheese, then a poached egg and finally, asparagus. Season with salt and pepper and serve immediately. (wheat, egg, milk)

23. **Poached egg with smoked salmon:** Ingredients: 1/4 cup butter, softened, 2 tablespoons fresh dill, 1 teaspoon lemon zest, 1 pinch cayenne pepper, salt and ground black pepper to taste, 1 teaspoon white vinegar, 1 pinch salt, 4 eggs, 2 English muffins, split and toasted, 4 ounces sliced smoked salmon, 1 pinch cayenne pepper, 4 small fresh dill sprig Stir butter, dill, lemon zest, cayenne pepper, salt, and black pepper in a bowl until combined. Set aside. Fill a large saucepan with 2.5-3 inches of water and bring to a boil over high heat. Reduce heat to medium-low; add vinegar and a pinch of salt. Crack an egg into a bowl then gently slip the egg into the water. Repeat with remaining eggs. Cook eggs until whites are firm and yolks have thickened but are not hard, 4-6 minutes. Remove eggs from water with a spoon, dab on a kitchen towel to remove excess water, and then transfer to a warm plate. Generously spread each English muffin half with dill butter. Top with a layer of smoked salmon, then 1 poached egg. Season with cayenne pepper, salt, and black pepper to taste. Garnish with a dill sprig and serve. (fish, egg, milk, wheat)

24. **Scrambled eggs with zucchini:** Ingredients: 4 eggs, lightly beaten, 2 tablespoons grated Parmesan cheese, 1-2 tablespoons olive oil, 1 zucchini, sliced 1/6- to 1/4-inch thick, garlic powder, or to taste, salt and ground black pepper to taste   Stir the eggs and Parmesan

cheese together in a bowl; set aside. Heat the olive oil in a large skillet over medium-high heat; cook the zucchini in the hot oil until softened and lightly browned, about 5-7 minutes. Season the zucchini with garlic powder, salt, and pepper. Reduce heat to medium; pour the egg mixture into the skillet. Cook, stirring gently, for about 2.5-3 minutes. Remove the skillet from the heat and cover. Keep covered off the heat until the eggs set, about 1.5-2 minutes more. (egg, milk)

Chicken

(Chicken breast should be the primary source of protein in a muscle building fitness diet. I recommend eating it every day)

25. **Spicy garlic-lime chicken:** Ingredients: 3/4 teaspoon salt, 1/4 teaspoon black pepper, 1/4 teaspoon cayenne pepper, 1/8 teaspoon paprika, 1/4 teaspoon garlic powder, 1/8 teaspoon onion powder, 1/4 teaspoon dried thyme, 1/4 teaspoon dried parsley, 4 boneless, skinless chicken breast halves, 2 tablespoons butter, 1 tablespoon olive oil, 2 teaspoons garlic powder, 3 tablespoons lime juice   In a small bowl, mix together salt, black pepper, cayenne, paprika, 1/4 teaspoon garlic powder, onion powder, thyme and parsley. Spice mixture should generously cover both sides of chicken breasts. Heat butter and olive oil in a large heavy skillet over medium heat. Sauté chicken until golden brown, about 6 minutes on each side. Sprinkle with 2 teaspoons garlic powder and lime juice. Cook 5-6 minutes more, stirring frequently to coat evenly with sauce. (milk)

26. **Easy and fast fitness chicken breast:** Ingredients: 4 skinless, boneless chicken breast halves, 2 tablespoons olive oil, 1 tablespoon sea salt, or to taste, 1 tablespoon water, or as

needed   Preheat convection oven to 390-400 degrees
F. Rub chicken breasts with olive oil and sprinkle both sides
with salt. Place chicken in a broiler pan. Bake in the
preheated oven for 10-12 minutes. Flip chicken and cook
until no longer pink in the center and the juices run clear,
about 15 minutes more. An instant-read thermometer
inserted into the center should read at least 165 degrees F.
Remove chicken from pan.

27. **Lemon-chicken:** Ingredients: 1 tbsp. cider vinegar, 1
    teaspoon mustard, 1 clove minced garlic, 1 tbsp. lemon
    juice, 1 teaspoon lime juice, 1 teaspoon brown sugar
    (optional) , salt and pepper to taste, 1 teaspoon olive oil, 2
    chicken breasts   In a large glass bowl, mix the cider
    vinegar, mustard, garlic, lime juice, lemon juice, brown
    sugar, salt, and pepper. Whisk in the olive oil. Place chicken
    in the mixture. Cover, and marinate for at least 8 hours, or
    overnight. Preheat an outdoor grill for high heat. Lightly oil
    the grill grate. Place chicken on the prepared grill, and cook
    6-8 minutes per side, until juices run clear. Discard
    marinade.

28. **Easy garlic-chicken:** Ingredients: 3 tablespoons butter, 4
    skinless, boneless chicken breast halves, 2 teaspoons garlic
    powder, 1 teaspoon seasoning salt, 1 teaspoon onion
    powder   Melt butter in a large skillet over medium
    high heat. Add chicken and sprinkle with garlic powder,
    seasoning salt and onion powder. Cook about 12-15 minutes
    on each side, or until chicken is cooked through and juices
    run clear. (milk)

29. **Grilled chicken breasts with grilled veggies:** Ingredients: 2
    chicken breasts, 3 bell peppers, 1 zucchini, salt and pepper
    to taste   Cut up peppers into big

chunks, and zucchini into big slices. Grill chicken and veggies over medium heat.(add olive oil if needed)

30. **Chicken breast teriyaki:** Ingredients: 4 skinless, boneless chicken breast halves, 1 cup teriyaki sauce, 1/4 cup lemon juice, 2 teaspoons minced fresh garlic, 2 teaspoons sesame oil   Place chicken, teriyaki sauce, lemon juice, garlic, and sesame oil in a large resalable plastic bag. Seal bag, and shake to coat. Place in refrigerator for 24 hours, turning every so often. Preheat grill for high heat. Lightly oil the grill grate. Remove chicken from bag, discarding any remaining marinade. Grill for 6 to 8 minutes each side, or until juices run clear when chicken is pierced with a fork. (soy)

31. **lemon-herb chicken:** Ingredients: 1 lemon, salt and pepper to taste, 1 tbsp. olive oil, 1 chicken breast, oregano to taste, parsley   Cut lemon in half, and squeeze juice from 1/2 lemon on chicken. Season with salt to taste. Let sit while you heat oil in a small skillet over medium low heat. When oil is hot, put chicken in skillet. As you sauté chicken, add juice from other 1/2 lemon, pepper to taste, and oregano. Sauté for 5 to 10 minutes each side, or until juices run clear. Serve with parsley for garnish.

32. **lettuce rolls:** Ingredients: 2tbsp olive oil, 2 half chicken breasts, ginger to taste, 1 tbsp. vinegar, 1 teaspoon honey, 1 tbsp. teriyaki sauce, 5 cherry tomatoes, 2 carrots, 2 green onions, bunch of almonds, lettuce leaf   Heat 1 tablespoon oil in a large skillet over medium-high heat. Sauté chicken and ginger in hot oil until chicken is cooked through, 7 to 10 minutes. Set aside. Whisk vinegar, teriyaki sauce, remaining 1 tablespoon oil, and honey together in a bowl. Add chicken mixture, cherries, carrots, green onion, and almonds; toss to combine. Spoon 1/12 the

chicken/cherry mixture onto the center of each lettuce leaf; roll leaf around filling and serve. (soy, tree nut)

33. **rosemary chicken breast:** Ingredients: 2 skinless, boneless chicken breasts, 2 cloves garlic, chopped, 2 tablespoons dried rosemary, 1 tablespoon lemon juice, salt and pepper to taste   Preheat oven to 380 degrees F .Cover the chicken breasts with garlic, then sprinkle with rosemary, lemon juice, and salt and pepper to taste. Place in a large baking dish and bake in the preheated oven for 25 minutes or until done and juices run clear (baking time will depend on the thickness of the chicken breasts).

Beef

(Should be grass-fed and lean.) I recommend eating it after workout)

34. **Beef and veggie stir-fry:** Ingredients: 3/4 pound beef round steak, 1/3 cup minced garlic, vegetables, red bell pepper (optional)   Cut beef steak lengthwise in half, then crosswise into thick strips. Add vegetables and 3 tablespoons water in large nonstick skillet. Cover and cook over medium-high heat 4-5 minutes or until crisp-tender. Remove and drain. Heat same pan over medium-high heat until hot. Add half of beef and half of garlic; stir-fry 1-2 minutes or until outside surface of beef is no longer pink. Remove. Repeat with remaining beef and garlic. Return all beef and vegetables to pan. Add stir-fry sauce and crushed red pepper; heat through. Serve over rice. (meat)

35. **beef with broccoli:** Ingredients: 1 pound round steak, thinly sliced into 2 inch pieces, 1 tbsp. olive oil, 1 broccoli   Heat

oil in large nonstick skillet over medium-high heat and cook steak, stirring frequently, 6 minutes or until almost done. Remove steak; keep warm. Add broccoli and continue cooking, stirring frequently, 4 minutes or until vegetables are tender. Add back steak and stir-fry sauce and cook, stirring frequently, 2-3 minutes or until heated through. Serve over prepared rice. (meat)

36. **marinated skirt steak:** Ingredients: 2/3 cup good quality red wine, 1/4 cup ketchup, 6 cloves garlic, minced, 2 teaspoons salt, 1 teaspoon dried rosemary, 1 teaspoon ground black pepper , 1 (1 1/2-pound) skirt steak, cut in half across the grain   Whisk wine, ketchup, garlic, kosher salt, rosemary, and black pepper together in a large bowl. Add skirt steak and turn to evenly coat. Cover the bowl with plastic wrap, and marinate in the refrigerator, 8 hours to overnight. Preheat an outdoor grill for high heat, and lightly oil the grate. Remove steak from marinade, shake off excess, and discard marinade. Cook steak on the preheated grill until meat shines, 3 to 4 minutes per side. An instant-read thermometer inserted into the center should read 130 degrees F (54 degrees C). Transfer meat to a plate and let rest for 5-7 minutes before slicing against the grain. (meat)

37. **garlic pepper steak:** Ingredients: 1 tablespoon olive oil , 2 cloves garlic, peeled and crushed, 1 tablespoon ground black pepper, 2 pounds round steak, 1 1/2 inches thick Preheat an outdoor grill for high heat and lightly oil grate. In a small bowl, mix together olive oil, garlic and pepper. Score steak and rub with the olive oil mixture. Place steak on the prepared grill. Cook 20-25 minutes, or to desired doneness, turning once. (meat)

38. beef salad: Ingredients: 2 green onions, chopped , 1 lemon grass, cut into 1 inch pieces, 1 cup chopped fresh cilantro, 1 cup chopped fresh mint leaves, 1 cup lime juice, 1/3 cup fish sauce, 1 tablespoon sweet chili sauce, 1/2 cup brown sugar (optional), 1 1/2 pounds steak fillet, 1 head leaf lettuce, 1/2 English cucumber, diced, 1 pint cherry tomatoes

In a large bowl, stir together the green onions, lemon grass, cilantro, mint leaves, lime juice, fish sauce, chili sauce and sugar until well combined and the sugar is dissolved. Adjust the flavor, if desired, by adding more sugar and/or fish sauce. Set aside. Cook the steak over high heat on a preheated grill for approximately 4-6 minutes on each side, until it is cooked medium. Do not overcook the meat! Remove from heat and slice into thin strips. Add the meat and its juices to the sauce and refrigerate, tightly covered, for at least 3 hours. Tear the lettuce into bite size pieces and place in a salad bowl. Arrange the cucumber on top of the lettuce, and then pour the meat and sauce over. Top with the cherry tomatoes and garnish with fresh cilantro leaves. (meat)

39. beef jerky: Ingredients: Worcestershire sauce , soy sauce, paprika, 1 teaspoon honey, 1 tbsp. onion powder, garlic powder, red pepper flakes, black pepper, 1 pound eye of round   Whisk Worcestershire sauce, soy sauce, paprika, honey, black pepper, red pepper flakes, garlic powder, and onion powder together. Add beef and turn to coat beef completely. Cover the bowl with plastic wrap and marinate in the fridge overnight. Preheat oven to 180 degrees F. Line a baking sheet with aluminum foil and place a wire rack over the foil. Transfer beef to paper towels to dry. Discard marinade. Arrange beef slices in a single layer on the prepared wire rack on the baking sheet. Bake beef until dry and leathery (3 to 4 hours). Cut into bite-size pieces. (meat, soy)

40. **Cuban steak:** Ingredients: 1/2 teaspoon cumin seeds , 1/3 cup orange juice , 2 tablespoons olive oil , 2 tablespoons steak seasoning, 1/4 teaspoons lime juice, 1/2 teaspoons dried oregano, 1 1/2 pounds beef rib-eye steaks

    Place cumin seeds into a small skillet over medium heat; stir constantly until seeds turn dark brown (about 1 minute). Immediately pour seeds into a bowl to stop the cooking. Mix cumin seeds with orange juice, olive oil, steak seasoning, lime juice, and oregano in a bowl. Place steaks into a large resalable plastic bag, pour orange juice marinade over the meat, and squeeze out air. Seal bag and turn it over several times to coat meat with marinade. Refrigerate for at least 30-40 minutes, or longer for extra flavor. Preheat an outdoor grill for medium-high heat and lightly oil the grate. Remove steaks from marinade, shaking off any excess. Discard used marinade. Grill steaks on the preheated grill until seared on the outsides and still slightly pink in the centers, 7-8 minutes per side. An instant-read meat thermometer inserted sideways into the center of the thickest steak should read 140 degrees F. Let steaks rest for 3 minutes before slicing. (meat)

41. **Tenderloin with herbs (not easy!):** Ingredients: 2 beef tenderloin steaks, 1/4 teaspoon salt, 1/2 teaspoon ground pepper, 2 tbsp. olive oil, 1 tablespoon unsalted butter, 2 tablespoons finely diced shallots , 1 tablespoon Dijon mustard, 1 tablespoon Worcestershire sauce, 2 tablespoons heavy cream, 2 teaspoons chopped fresh parsley, 1 teaspoon chopped fresh chives , 1 teaspoon chopped fresh oregano   Preheat oven to 430 degrees F. Pat the steaks dry with paper towels; season both sides with salt

and pepper. Allow steaks to rest at room temperature for about 40 minutes while the oven pre-heats. Heat a 10-inch cast iron pan over medium-high heat for about one minute. Add the oil to pan and swirl to evenly distribute the oil. Place the steaks in the pan, allowing place between. Cook without turning steaks for 2-2.5 minutes, and then flip the steaks over. The steaks should release easily, without sticking to the pan. Immediately place cast iron pan into the hot oven. Cook steaks until firm and reddish-pink and juicy in the center, about 7 minutes. An instant-read thermometer inserted into the center should read 130 degrees F (54 degrees C). Remove skillet from oven and transfer steaks to a warm plate lightly tented with foil. (The internal temperature of the steaks will increase by about 5 degrees while resting.) Melt butter in the same skillet over low heat; add diced shallots. Cook and stir, releasing the browned bits from the bottom of the pan, about 1 minute. Stir in the mustard. Increase the heat to medium-high. Whisk in Worcestershire sauce, continuing to scrape up browned bits from the pan. Bring to a boil and cook until slightly reduced, about 5 minutes. Reduce the heat to medium. Whisk in the cream; simmer until sauce clings to the back of a spoon, about 2 minutes. Stir in the parsley, chives, and oregano. Spoon the herb sauce over steaks; serve immediately. (meat, milk)

42. **steak salad:** Ingredients: 1 3/4 pounds beef sirloin steak , 1/3 cup olive oil , 3 tablespoons red wine vinegar , 2 tablespoons lemon juice , 1 clove garlic, minced, 1/2 teaspoon salt, 1/8 teaspoon ground black pepper, 1 teaspoon Worcestershire sauce , 3/4 cup crumbled blue cheese, 8 cups lettuce - rinsed, dried, and torn into bite-size pieces, 2 tomatoes, sliced, 1 small green bell pepper, sliced,

1 carrot, sliced, 1/2 cup sliced red onion

Preheat grill for high heat. Lightly oil grate. Place steak on grill and cook for 3 to 5 minutes per side or until desired doneness is reached. Remove from heat and let sit until cool enough to handle. Slice steak into bite size pieces. In a small bowl, whisk together the olive oil, vinegar, lemon juice, garlic, salt, pepper and Worcestershire sauce. Mix in the cheese. Cover and place dressing in refrigerator. Onto chilled plates arrange the lettuce, tomato, pepper and onion. Top with steak and drizzle with dressing. Serve with crusty grilled bread. (meat, milk)

Seafood

(Although it is not as popular as chicken, it contains very high amount of protein)

43. **spicy grilled shrimp:** Ingredients: 1 clove garlic minced, salt, 1/2 teaspoon cayenne pepper , 1 teaspoon paprika , 1 tablespoon olive oil(add more if it is needed), 2 pounds large shrimp, peeled and deveined , 1 tablespoon lemon juice
Preheat grill for medium heat. In a small bowl, mix the garlic with the salt. Mix in cayenne pepper and paprika, and then stir in olive oil and lemon juice to form a paste. In a large bowl, toss shrimp with garlic paste until fully coated. Lightly oil grill grate. Cook shrimp for 2.5-3 minutes per side, or until opaque. Transfer to a serving dish and serve. (shellfish)

44. **butter-garlic shrimp:** Ingredients: 1 tablespoon olive oil, 1 pound shrimp, peeled and deveined, salt, 5-6 cloves garlic, minced, 1/4 teaspoon red pepper flakes, 2.5 tablespoons lemon juice, 1/2 teaspoons butter, parsley
Heat olive oil in a heavy skillet over high heat. Place shrimp in an even layer on the bottom of the pan and cook for 1

minute without stirring. Season shrimp with salt; cook and stir until shrimp begin to turn pink, about 1 minute. Add garlic and red pepper flakes; cook with stirring for 1 minute. Stir in lemon juice, 1 1/2 teaspoon cold butter, and parsley. Cook until butter has melted, about 1 minute, and then turn heat to low. Cook and stir until all shrimps are pink and opaque, about 2 to 3 minutes. Remove shrimp with a spoon and transfer to a bowl; continue to cook sauce, adding water 1 teaspoon at a time if too thick, about 2 minutes. Season with salt to taste. Serve shrimp topped with the pan sauce. Garnish with remaining flat-leaf parsley if needed. (shellfish, milk)

45. **Sesame shrimp stir-fry:** Ingredients: 2 cups water, 1 cup uncooked white rice, 1 tablespoon sesame oil, 1 clove garlic, minced, 1 teaspoon ground ginger, 1/4 teaspoon cayenne pepper, 1 tablespoon sesame seed, ground black pepper, 1 bell pepper, 3 tablespoons teriyaki sauce, 3 onions, 1 pound peas, 1/8 cup cornstarch, salt   In a medium saucepan, bring water to a boil and add salt. Add rice, reduce heat, cover and simmer for about 20 minutes. While rice is simmering, combine shrimp, ginger, cayenne pepper, garlic, sesame seeds and black pepper in a large plastic food storage bag. Allow to marinate in the refrigerator. Heat some sesame oil in a large wok. Add red bell pepper and onions; sauté 3 to 4 minutes to soften slightly. Add teriyaki sauce. Add peas and shrimp with seasoning; sauté 4 minutes or until shrimp are opaque. Stir cornstarch into to wok; cook, stirring until mixture boils. Sprinkle with salt. Spoon shrimp mixture over rice. (shellfish, soy, corn)

46. **Mexican shrimp:** Ingredients: 1 pound shrimp, peeled and deveined, 1 tablespoon olive oil, 2 teaspoons tequila, 3

tablespoons chopped fresh cilantro, 2 tablespoons fresh lime juice, 2 cloves garlic, minced, 1/4 teaspoon cayenne pepper, salt   Stir shrimp, olive oil, cilantro, lime juice, garlic, tequila, cayenne pepper, and salt together in a bowl. Cover the bowl with plastic wrap and refrigerate shrimp in marinade for at least 30 minutes. Preheat an outdoor grill for high heat and lightly oil grate. Remove shrimp from bowl and thread onto skewers; discard used marinade. Cook on the preheated grill until shrimp turn pink, 2 to 3 minutes per side. (shellfish)

47. **spicy lime grilled shrimp:** Ingredients: 1 pound shrimp, peeled and deveined, 1/3 teaspoon Cajun pepper, 1 teaspoon lime juice, 1 tablespoon olive oil,
Mix together the Cajun pepper , lime juice, and olive oil in a resalable plastic bag. Add the shrimp, coat with the marinade, squeeze out excess air, and seal the bag. Marinate in the fridge for at least 30 minutes. Preheat an outdoor grill for medium heat, and lightly oil the grate. Remove the shrimp from the marinade. Discard the used marinade. Cook the shrimp on the preheated grill until they are bright pink on the outside and the meat is no longer transparent in the center, about 2 minutes per side. (shellfish)

48. **shrimp salad:** Ingredients: 1 pound previously cooked deveined and peeled shrimp, 1 cup chopped celery , 1 large carrot , 2 hard-cooked eggs, ½ cup mayonnaise, salt and pepper to taste   In a large bowl, mix the shrimp, celery, carrot(shredded), eggs, and mayonnaise. Season with salt and pepper. Chill until ready to serve. (shellfish, egg)

(It should be filling and it can contain a bit more fat or sugar than the rest of your meals)

(*I am not going in detail with these because they are really simple)

49. **Spinach and cheese stuffed omelet (**egg, milk**):**
Beat eggs, a drop of milk, salt and pepper in small bowl until blended. Heat butter in 7 to 10-inch nonstick omelet pan or skillet over medium-high heat until hot. Pour in the egg mixture. Mixture should set immediately at edges.
Push cooked portions from edges toward the center with inverted turner so that uncooked eggs can reach the hot pan surface. Continue cooking, tilting pan and gently moving cooked portions. When top surface of eggs is thickened and no visible liquid egg remains, Put some spinach leaves and cheese of your choice on one side of the
omelet. Fold omelet in half with turner. With a quick flip of the wrist, turn pan and slide omelet onto
plate. Serve immediately.

50. **Two eggs mixed with two bananas and made as pancakes (aka banana pancake):** (egg) Combine flour, white sugar, baking powder and salt. In a separate bowl, mix together egg, milk, vegetable oil and bananas. Stir flour mixture into banana mixture; batter will be slightly lumpy. Heat a lightly oiled griddle or frying pan over medium high heat. Pour or scoop the batter onto the griddle, using approximately 1/4 cup for each pancake. Cook until pancakes are golden brown on both sides; serve hot.

51. **Oats with plain Greek yoghurt with banana slices on top** (milk)**:** Pour some plain Greek yoghurt and 1 cup of oats in a bowl, mix the ingredients. Slice up a banana and place it on top.

52. **Toast of whole-grain bread with avocado and cherry-tomatoes on it** (wheat): Take 2 avocados and toast a thin slice from whole-grain bread. Cut cherry tomatoes in half. Cut your avocados in half, remove the pit, scoop the flesh into a bowl or onto the side of your plate, and mash it up with a fork. Place the mashed avocado on top on the slice of toast, season it with some salt and add some cherry tomatoes.

53. **Oatmeal seasoned with cinnamon and baked slices of apple on top:** Preheat the oven to 375 degrees. Grease a 9-inch square baking dish. In a medium mixing bowl, combine the oats, cinnamon, baking powder, salt and nutmeg. Whisk to combine. In a smaller mixing bowl, combine the milk, maple syrup or honey, egg, half of the butter or coconut oil, and vanilla. Whisk until blended. Mix the two. Pour the oatmeal mixture over the baking dish and spread evenly. Bake for 40-45 minutes, until the top is golden and the oats are set. Slice some apples on top.

54. **Strawberry and banana smoothie:** Place a bunch of strawberry and a frozen banana into the blender pitcher. Cover with lid and tamper (if your blender comes with one). Start at a low speed and increase incrementally. If your blender doesn't have a tamper, you might need to blend in stages while turning off and readjusting ingredients with a spoon and relending. Add water or milk as needed and blend until smooth. Pour and serve immediately.

55. **Blueberry, banana, red berry smoothie (add yoghurt/milk/water if needed)** Put 1 frozen banana, a bunch of blueberry and red berry into the blender pitcher Cover with lid and tamper. Start at a low speed and increase incrementally Add water or milk as needed and blend until smooth. Pour and serve immediately.

56. **Almond, banana and cinnamon smoothie (water/yoghurt/milk)** (tree nut) Put 1 frozen banana, a bunch of roasted almond and a pinch of cinnamon into the blender pitcher. Cover with lid and tamper. Start at a low speed and increase incrementally Add water or milk as needed and blend until smooth. Pour and serve immediately.

57. **Oats, blueberry and roasted almonds with Greek yoghurt** (tree nut, milk) Pour some plain Greek yoghurt, a bunch of roasted almonds, some blueberry and 1 cup of oats in a bowl, mix the ingredients. Enjoy your meal.

58. **Oatmeal with milk and honey (cinnamon is optional)** (milk) Take **1/2 cup oats to 1 cup of water, milk or combination of both**. Then place in the microwave without a cover on it. Microwave on high for 2 minutes and the consistency should be perfect. Pour some honey on top and enjoy.

59. **Fruit of any kind and just a little bit (!)**

60. **Baked oatmeal with banana and almond/peanut butter on top** (tree nut/peanut)**:** Preheat the oven to 375 degrees. Grease a 9-inch square baking dish. In a medium mixing bowl, combine the oats, almonds/peanut butter, baking powder, salt and nutmeg. Whisk to combine. In a smaller mixing bowl, combine the milk, maple syrup or honey, egg, half of the butter or coconut oil, and vanilla. Whisk until blended. Mix the two. Pour the oatmeal mixture over the baking dish and spread evenly. Bake for 40-45 minutes, until the top is golden and the oats are set. Slice some bananas on top.

61. **Baked oatmeal with blueberry and apple in it:** Preheat the oven to 375 degrees. Grease a 9-inch square baking dish. In a medium mixing bowl, combine the oats, cinnamon, baking powder, salt and nutmeg. Whisk to combine. In a smaller mixing bowl, combine the milk, maple syrup or honey, egg, half of the butter or coconut oil, and vanilla. Whisk until blended. Mix the two. Place some blueberry in the dish. Pour the oatmeal mixture over the baking dish and spread evenly. Bake for 40-45 minutes, until the top is golden and the oats are set. Slice some apples on top.

Pre-workout:

You should eat something easier to digest before workout. I highlighted those on the list with green. But you shouldn't eat protein packed foods with heavy carbs because together it messes up your stomach! It is also very important that the meal should contain protein, fiber, carbohydrate. Fruit is also great to be eaten before workout due to its fructose which gives you energy. But the most important of all is coffee. It helps you getting more concentrated, provides easier mind-muscle connection and helps fat loss.

After workout:

The 30 minute mark is not real! So nothing happens when you do not eat protein within 30 mins after the workout. It is a myth. But you can give yourself a bit fatter than you would normally. Nothing special besides that, you should eat the regular amount of protein and carbs after workout.

*allergy warnings are marked with red